The
30
Year Diet:

The Journey of Me, Fat Girl and My FOPA

Robin L. Nutter

Important Notice from the author, Robin L. Nutter

This book is dedicated to my family who has supported me through every difficult struggle. The love of family makes me a better daughter, aunt, friend and wife. The joy of being a mother gives me the strength to continue to push through the obstacles of life and bring my inner strengths to the surface. And to my husband that encouraged me to put my thoughts on paper and never lets me forget our love is always and forever.

- Robin Nutter

As I write this I'm in awe and truly touched by her strength and courage. She is sharing her struggles and triumphs through pain and laughter. It's a testament to her giving spirit. And I'm happy to encourage you to read this book and follow her journey of thirty years of dieting. What I like most about The Thirty Year Diet is her openness and candor. Her story is personal and poignant, relatable, engaging, empowering, and hilariously funny. I love that she can face her failures with strength, and humor fall down and get right back up and continue her endless battle with Fat Girl and her FOPA. She teaches us all that we all are truly beautiful.

-Your loving daughter, Cristina Nutter

TABLE OF CONTENTS

INTRODUCTION

Here's the thing. I'm not fat but I have a Fat Girl taking up residence in my head. She's been there since I was 9 years old. Over the decades, we've developed a love-hate relationship.

I hate when she tells me that I look fat in my jeans; that no one loves me; or that success will only present itself after I lose weight. But the love I have for her is equally strong. I love her creative ways of getting rid of my doughnut—the mushy circle of fat that decorates my belly button.

My doughnut has acquired many names over the years, depending on my clothing size and the number on the scale. I've called it "my daughter's old apartment," "my muffin top," "my cootchie cover," "spare tire," "love handles," and currently as my "FOPA" (otherwise known as the Fat Over Private Area).

Fat Girl's voice is boisterous and confident. She provides me with endless ways to conquer and defeat the weight by tirelessly researching techniques and methods on the Internet, watching commercials, investigating infomercials, and getting ideas through word of mouth.

I'll spell out how she got there but the bottom line is that she's taken me on a journey to places only few have been and pushed me to try things that have made me ask the question, "Did I really take myself there?"

I did some things you might have done. Diets, fads and techniques that either made me laugh or resulted in secrets that I should take to my grave.

I let my Fat Girl determine how I loved, whether it was me or someone else. She determined my relationships, career paths, and several life choices that I've made over the past 34 years.

How? By letting her feed me all sorts of negative thoughts that only brought me down and made me feel like I was nothing. But no more! I'm breaking free and I want you to join me.

Whatever you call that special part of you that causes frustration, I want you to point to it, call it by name, wrap your hands around it, shake it and say, "its okay if you never leave. I WILL love myself no matter what."

I have been on a nearly four-decade-long journey (also called the never-ending-diet plan), believing that mythical idea that if I could lose just 10, or 20, or 30, or even 40 pounds, my life would be perfect.

I would get a better job, fall in love, and lay on the beach in a two-piece bikini…stretch-mark-free with 8-pack abs, and breasts as perky as Halle Berry's in a James Bond movie.

But honestly, the number on the scale really didn't matter unless it was a number I liked—because the weight I lost was never good enough.

So after spending a good $20,000 (money I didn't have, by the way) on unrealistic weight-loss ventures and pushing my body to its physical limit, I was left with a badly bruised self-image, a compromised digestive system, depression, anxiety disorders, and a tremendous amount of dissatisfaction with my life.

CHAPTER 1

Now, this is not a story about defeat. It's a story about overcoming and empowerment. We shouldn't let our so-called flaws define us like I did in the past.

Instead, this book is meant to be an empathetic trip down memory lane that hopefully will help you see how the search for happiness and acceptance can lead any of us to exclusively and obsessively focusing on our weight—when our weight isn't even the issue!

It's a way for you to learn how your weight, your diet, or your looks don't have to define the incredible spirit and potential joy within you. Be honest, you're letting how you feel in those jeans or how your butt looks in a dressing room mirror determine your moods and decisions—in ways you don't even realize.

It's okay if you don't believe me. I didn't believe it for the longest time either. In fact, I did things in the quest for a slim body that some would say is a borderline addiction to dieting, but I never viewed it that way.

That is, not until I had consumed a combination of digestive enzymes and diet pills that caused me to break out in a horrendous rash and run to the ER with heart-attack-like symptoms.

After years of self-abuse, I learned from my doctor that my body couldn't tolerate any more diet or appetite-suppressant pills. In fact, those pills didn't affect my weight at all.

I've consumed over-the-counter pills, under-the-counter pills, liquids, solids, powders, gel tabs, capsules, time release tablets, and 24-hour appetite suppressants… you name it. I've swallowed it, rubbed it on my body, meditated it into fruition, and squeezed my ass into it…all in the name of pursing my perfect self-image.

And the funny thing about it all is that I'm not overweight! Or even slightly obese! I'm a 40ish mother (5'4 and 153 pounds) who just can't get rid of that little bit of 23-year-old baby weight around my stomach from my beautiful daughter.

You know what I'm talking about—that little bulge around your belly button. The jelly-like, cellulite-filled fat that you would stand in a line wrapping around three blocks all day if there was a doctor giving away free tummy tucks.

For you, it might mean getting rid of that extra fat underneath your chin, pimply skin, or thin hair.

It's basically whatever you stare at in mirror that you just don't like about yourself. Or maybe it's nothing at all… just all in your mind. That something only visible to you and no one else.

How long have you looked at this one aspect of your body and thought life will be so much better as soon as I remove my fatal flaw?

What would happen if, instead, you appreciated that one thing you zoned in on every time you looked in the mirror? Or better yet, what if you focused on the millions of other attributes staring back at you in the mirror? The best of you.

CHAPTER 2

Now, I'm not saying don't keep working hard to improve yourself. I think that's part of our time here on earth.

But is self-improvement always a physical quest?

Aren't there other things you could learn about yourself spiritually, emotionally, and mentally? Wouldn't it be nice to generate greater self-insight? That might even foster the right kind of mindset to lose weight and keep it off permanently.

You could do all of this right now by taking a moment to look in the mirror and appreciate the lovely creature looking back at you. That's a very difficult task that has taken me years to attempt and it takes a continuous amount of effort today.

Ladies, we are beautiful in all of our unique shapes, and it is our responsibility and privilege to take care of ourselves—so that we can be the amazing women our Creator meant for us to be. Be a better you, for yourself, your family, and for others.

Yet, as with everything in life, there is a thin line between taking care of us and careening off into a dangerous descent. There are so many things you can do to be healthy.

In spite of the abuse I've put myself through I'm actually in better health than you would think…except for the mental battle I fight with my weight.

That's where Fat Girl came into existence. She is the Fat Girl who feeds me negativity and a formidable foe.

She sounds made up but she's as real in my mind as logic, facts, and knowledge. I've nurtured and loved her for most of my life because even though we fight I know she loves me too.

I have a difficult time remembering the "me" before my diet journey. But when I do think of that "old me," all I can do is smile and shake my head.

The "old me" had a free spirit, a type of youthful innocence. The little girl everyone wanted to be around. But after a small mean bite of negativity, the "old me" desired self-deprecation and my newly emerged Fat Girl was more than obliged to give it.

I let Fat Girl hold me back from experiencing new things, being spontaneous, and most of all creating a regret-free life. What is your so-called "logical" brain holding you back from? Developing great relationships? Giving it your all in your career? Living your life?

A few simple words that may seem so innocent to most people, started my dieting journey, and an innocent 9-year-old was forever changed by a few choice words.

CHAPTER 3

So I'm 9 years old and standing on the landing of my parents' house in suburban Ohio. It's Sunday evening and we've just had a family meal.

I had plans for playing a neighborhood kickball game

that evening. But I was wondering why my siblings were looking at me and laughing.

I didn't quite understand it but I felt so embarrassed. I thought to myself, "Are they talking to me?" I looked at each of my siblings in confusion.

I remember blinking my eyes like I was waking up from a dream. I can still hear their words loud and clear. "You have to come back and wash the dishes, Miss Piggy!" "Hey, you fat girl, come down and help clean up."

That's it. Just two sentences dramatically changed my life and how I looked at myself. And it all started out like any other Sunday.

For our family, it was a morning rush for the one bathroom in the house that was shared by my parents, four older sisters, and younger brother. We all knew the order of importance. Daddy goes first.

My father (a church deacon and leader of the men's choir) hated to be late for any event. I can still smell the burn from the pressing comb in the air from the night before, mixing with the aroma of the tasty scrambled egg sandwich that was on the dining room table for my father's breakfast.

This man ran a tight ship: Good grades were a must. If you didn't like the rules it was "his shack, Jack," and you could get out. He was a man of many words and gestures that still echo throughout our small town— long after he died of cancer several years ago.

My father was the lead vocalist in the male choir, handled the church's collection plate, confirmed the pastor's speech with a hearty "Amen," visited the sick and shut-in, and made sure he was back home in time for Sunday dinner and football.

That was my father's Sunday ritual, which in turn was our family ritual. This particular Sunday, my father invited the pastor and his family over for dinner. I was excited because we all admired the pastor's three sons. They were little pastors in training, with their father's personality, handsome smiles, and lots of swagger.

I had my eye, even at 9, on the middle one—not too old for me and not a mama's boy. This kid knew he was cute. He talked to every girl in the church, except for my best friend Dee. She said his armpits smelled like vomit, but I didn't care. In my mind, he was going to be my husband and I was going to be the mother of the church.

My mom served the traditional Baptist Sunday dinner of fried chicken, collard greens, macaroni and cheese (baked of course), with big buttery dinner rolls and a large pitcher of Kool-Aid. After dinner, the men retreated to the TV room while the women gossiped about church and the members that weren't there while sitting on the front porch.

And the kids cleared the table. Back then, there wasn't a chore list on the refrigerator or a false eagerness to clean for a weekly allowance. It was understood: Before playtime, or really any free time, there was chore time.

Every room was your room and your responsibility. But I had it planned out: Dinner, change out of my church clothes, bathroom break, clear the table, and then the big kickball game!

Finally, we were done. I stood up from the table and headed upstairs to wash my hands. My mind was focused on whose team I would be on, if the girls next door were finished with their dinner, if the kids across the street would join in, and, of course, if the pastor's sons would join us.

I was happy, carefree, and couldn't wait to go play. Little did I know that would be the last time I felt such innocence and pure happiness.

"You have to come back here and wash the dishes, Miss Piggy!" "Did you hear me, Shamu!!?!"

With a smirk on her face, my sister was yelling at me but I didn't understand. The tone of her voice sounded so demeaning and ugly. I thought these names were great.

Everyone loves to go on a family trip and see Shamu at Sea World; any kid would love to see Shamu splashing the visitors in the stands. Plus, who didn't love The Muppet Show? Miss Piggy was awesome. She wore ball gowns and a tiara. Even Kermit loved her.

Still, I stood there with tears in my eyes, processing

my thoughts with disbelief and confusion. The names meant so much to me but the way I felt was horrible. Darkness overwhelmed me.

My life was no longer the life I knew. Daddy's little girl—who used to hide waiting for her father to come home from work, dance around in the kitchen, and happily hold out a plate waiting to be served—was gone.

If I had only known the meaning of true self-worth, confidence, and inner joy, those hurtful comments from my immature sister would have rolled off my back. I would have given her a perfect 9-year-old comeback and went on my merry way to play kickball with my friends.

But I was only 9. Instead, I raced up to my room to cry as those words scalded a negative image of me in my mind. Those few words gave birth to Fat Girl. They also started a mental and physical battle that can only be compared with an apocalyptic world war.

Sometimes, it's seemingly little events that have the biggest impact on our lives. Decades after, even when it has no hold, these events still drive our entire way of thinking and being.

What was it for you? An embarrassing moment at school? Being snubbed by the cool kids? Or hearing to your face that you weren't good enough?

It stings, doesn't it? It might even make you cringe to relive that event years later...the emotions are still fresh in your mind as if it happened yesterday.

Don't worry; the power of these painful memories will fade if you learn how to redirect your thoughts. But for me, that didn't happen until after I had put myself through a litany list of diets, workouts, weight-loss tricks, and other gimmicks.

Fat Girl sought to recreate me into the ideal women who had it all. As the tears saturated my pillow, Fat Girl began feeding and sending me pessimistic thoughts.

She planted harsh mental images and taught me how to surround myself with adversity, making me believe that this tornado of pain would always be my life. I learned to apply those words to my body parts and hate them. Instead of food, I consumed negativity.

My womanly curves became my huge bulge. My stomach morphed into my FOPA that fueled endless complaints of having to tuck my stomach into my pants.

The battle between Fat Girl and I raged on to eradicate my FOPA. It was a quest for a perfect self-image…skinny, happy and unstoppable with the help of Fat Girl.

CHAPTER 4

After that fateful dinner scene, I would spend the next few, formative years of my life focusing on my weight and how I needed to be thinner—so that everyone would love me and, most importantly, so that I would start to love myself.

Rather than challenge the authority of my sister, or

anyone else, who taunted me about my looks, I accepted their comments and welcomed the self-deprecation. I didn't do anything dramatic action-wise, but inwardly, the words had set off a cataclysmic impact on my self-image.

Suddenly, I was uncomfortable in my body. I felt ugly and fat. I carried all of those emotions deep within my soul.

As countless others have done, I started to become the kid who made everyone laugh, masking my self-hatred. As long as others were happy and laughing at my quirky sense of humor, they weren't paying attention to my flaws or making comments about my looks.

I felt comfort in knowing I could beat others to the punch when it came to insults. It became much easier to demean my curves and make jokes about how I looked. But while I laughed along with others, I was hurting and hating myself.

The negative words from Fat Girl echoed in my head—like "How could you possible feel good with all that weight?" and "You have to lose that disgusting bulge"—became more comfortable and started to fit me. The words were me, and I was them.

I became the ugliness that dark persona. The negative words and insults repeated themselves over and over. I fed off that negativity until I had a belly full of self-hate. That was the fuel that gave me a perverted type of justice to fight.

I decided I was never going to be called "fat" again by anyone but me. And Fat Girl was going to lead me to the land of skinny!!

It's not like I started getting into fights with my classmates but mentally I fed myself with those provocative thoughts, and I never stopped. I had constant thoughts about my appearance and how it could be better. So with a rapid acceptance that my life would only improve when I lowered the number on the scale, at 12 I started looking for methods to control my weight.

The first weight machine I ever saw was that ridiculous one that claimed it would shake the weight off of you. It was big in the 1970's and it promised to shake the fat off your waist and hips (or at least that's what I thought it would do).

I'm sure some of you ladies remember strapping yourself in, pushing the start button, and watching every inch of cellulite shake uncontrollably. I remember it vividly. I remember trying it and thinking this is it! It's so easy and I'll be thin before you know it.

A little shake here, a little shake there, and "voila," I'm thin! Little did I know this would be the first of many feelings of disappointment by believing that just one method or technique could erase all my flaws and create self-happiness. I remember trying it. It was fun but ineffective.

The concept of a weight machine shaking flab off is similar to any quick weight-loss method out there in the diet industry, especially for women. If we see something working for even one woman, we're willing to give it a try.

I enjoy watching the advertisements for weight-loss workouts and the promises of instant success. I get the same feelings of this-is-the-one weight-loss gratification as I did when I was 12, staring at the huge stomach band on the fat-shaking machine.

Since I didn't really have many weight-loss options at 12, I resorted to starvation, which I simply saw as fasting. When you're younger and you don't eat regularly for a couple of days, "POOF," you lose weight. I used to eat little to nothing for a few days and I got away with it.

No one noticed if I skipped breakfast during our hectic mornings with everyone rushing out the door. No one saw me focusing on conversations rather than a sandwich at lunch. And since we didn't always sit down together as a family for dinner during the week, I could get away with not eating much dinner.

I can remember my brother and I were usually the last at the dinner table, so it was easy to dump most of my food in the closet underneath the stairs. I'm really surprised after all these years no one ever noticed the smell of rotting food in the family dining room.

However, missing a meal when you're younger is much different than missing a meal in your 40's. Your body will switch to starvation mode and start storing fat. Like a squirrel storing nuts for the winter.

You may think by missing a meal you'll be able to get into those jeans over the weekend but we've all heard the screams from our jeans, begging to be placed back in the "when-I-lose-the-weight" section of your closet.

Those were the good 'ole days of dieting; cheap, easy and fast.

But as puberty and hormones began to transform my body into yet another unwelcoming shape, I (with the help of Fat Girl) began to think of new ways to drastically improve my weight-loss regime: Something more effective and quick that could stop the hunger cravings altogether.

A magic pill or elixir that would give me a slim body in a snap. So Fat Girl and I decided appetite suppressants were the key to opening the weight-loss door and taking us to the wondrous land of skinny!!!

CHAPTER 5

Fat Girl and I were like thieves in the night, conjuring up ideas on how to find ways to get the fat off (aka, acquire the goods to lose the weight). At first, it was a cloak-and-dagger mission.

I would go to the local pharmacy and get some over-the-counter diet pills or diuretics and stash them in my secret hiding place: inside the pocket of the ugliest winter coat I had. I would sneak them and they worked. "Eureka!"

That was in the days of high metabolism. I could pop a couple pills in my mouth and my fast-acting metabolism would take care of the rest. Directions? I don't need no stinking directions! If one works, Fat Girl confirmed two work great!!!

What's funny is while my mind focused on my weight it seemed at all times—in my dreams, when I woke up, as I brushed my teeth, on the drive home from school or to friends' houses—I don't remember ever telling my friends, family, or anyone else about my weight obsession or Fat Girl.

For example, my best friend Dee didn't know what was happening. She was the epitome of the classic cheerleader: pencil-thin frame and perky little boobs. She wore those annoyingly tiny bloomers and tight little tops. She had great legs and a perfect smile.

And to top it off, she ate anything she wanted (burgers, fries, pizza, sweets, Italian, Asian, Soul Food), without gaining a pound!

I was also a cheerleader and on the basketball team, with a fairly toned and trim body as I reflect back on it. Short, athletic, and firm. Oh! To have that butt again! Those were the good 'ole days of youthful skin full of elasticity and plump collagen!

But I never let Dee in on what Fat Girl was forcing me into until many, many years later. In fact, after I let her in on what I had been doing (poor thing), all I discussed with her was weight control. Finally, someone I could talk to and tell what this fat little bitch had been doing to me!!

Before adding Dee to the mix it was just me and Fat Girl, on this mission for a still undefined, but perfect, weight. I began to use my weight as the scapegoat for any disappointment in my life.

Sure, I was in the homecoming court, on the dance team, and a fun cheerleader. But like in most schools, popularity was huge, and any slight rejection or snub had me reinforcing in my mind that I had to be disciplined and stern about my weight and image.

You probably don't need this spelled out, but let me just note that peer pressure is a BITCH. I'm sure some of you have been ridiculed by classmates, friends, or even your family members. It can and sometimes will drive you to the edge. Peer-pressure can take you to dark places that will lead you to negative thoughts, and deeds that you think will rid you of the pain. Or, you lose your mind for a brief moment to create a Fat Girl in your head.

I gave into peer-pressure as I got older and drank with friends. I found alcohol to be an effective appetite suppressant. And the added benefit was it dealt with Fat Girl.

The more I drank, the less she talked about my fat thighs. The more she laughed and enjoyed the alcohol, the less she told me I'm worthless. Oh, and she enjoyed the munchies. She loved to eat as much as I do. In fact, she encouraged it. So much so that she told me White Castle was where we were born.

With alcohol, I felt free from the ridicule and pressure to be skinny for just one night. But then with the rise of the sun, so came the rise of Fat Girl, who forgot how much fun she had the night before. She blamed me for having no self-control and eating shit. She told me that I deserved to be sick...and now she had to throw up.

She made me pay until I stepped on the scale and showed her how much weight I'd lost from being dehydrated from the alcohol in my system. When I stepped on the scale, she was elated with joy and so was I that those two pounds lost from dehydration had shut her up until the next weigh-in.

There were headaches, hangovers, and vomiting to contend with, but adding some alcohol in the mix let me drink more calories and eat less. But that didn't last long because I got tired of feeling nauseous, worn-down, dizzy, and pretending that I remembered how much fun I had.

I made it through high school and was whisked to Florida to go to college. I was out of Ohio and in the big city of Miami. Miami was the land of the tight and fit by any means necessary. Whether the fat was sucked out or sweated out, the pressure to be thin was on again.

Me and Fat Girl were about to get into a bikini and

cause cars to crash while turning every head on South Beach. It didn't turn out that way. Before the cars crashed and heads turned on South Beach, I was 20 and pregnant with my one, and only, daughter.

Surprisingly, I did not worry one bit about my weight during the pregnancy. I gave up smoking and alcohol of any and all kinds, and began eating regularly, ignoring Fat Girl for the first time in years.

But sometimes, I indulged a bit. Maybe I indulged a bit too much. I enjoyed every morsel of pizza, rice crispy treat, and jar of peanut butter I could get my hands on. If it wasn't nailed down, I ate it.

I became a victim to that popular myth that I'm "eating for two," and the baby weight would somehow magically dissolve before I left the hospital. I even took smaller pre-maternity clothes with me, which turned out to be wasteful packing. It was a choice between wearing home the hospital gown or maternity clothes. Needless to say, I chose the maternity clothes.

I learned the hard way that the weight doesn't come off right after childbirth. It was a shock and Fat Girl was right there shaking that fat little finger in my face saying, "I told you so!"

She was more determined than ever to get me back on the slimmed-down bandwagon. But she told me I needed more than just appetite suppressants. It was time for the big guns.

Despite using OTC diet aids in high school, I wasn't

much of a pill taker. But I was raising a child on my own, working full time, and attending college classes. I didn't have the energy, time, or discipline to do this the all-natural way, or with some cheap, caffeine-filled caplet.

Fat Girl was about to take me to the diet-pill promise land! It was time to pull up my big-girl panties and ride the prescription train to Skinnyland!

So I went to my doctor and asked for prescription-strength help. This is around the time that diet prescription drugs were the big craze among women wanting to fight the bulge. The magic pills were flooding the market and trumpeted as big successes.

I took a prescription magic pill that allowed me to eat whatever my heart desired, while still having the weight come off. It wasn't as strong as the prescriptions that were killing people but it had some serious side effects…like dizziness, dry mouth, insomnia, and constipation.

I was prescribed a sleeping pill to help me sleep, a laxative for the constipation, and told to drink plenty of water. Fat Girl was in fat-free heaven. But I feared this little obesity pill, even while I took it.

I would call my mom, who then knew I was a bit weight-obsessed, and told her, "I'm taking this pill. If anything happens and you get a call from the hospital, make sure to tell the paramedics to look in my purse."

To actually believe that I could die while taking this

prescription drug and doing it anyway because I wanted to look trim tells you that Fat Girl was in full control of my priorities, health, and life.

Don't get me wrong. I did everything in my power to be a good parent to my daughter and never let her know the pressure I felt to lose weight and my quest to have the perfect body.

There were plenty of secrets in my closet that I have long since emptied. One of those secrets was my need to medicate my extra pounds away for good. Keep in mind that my weight fluctuated from 135 to 140 pounds at the time.

I was no way obese or overweight. But it didn't matter. Fat Girl said I needed to take the pills. They were working, so I took the pills. If I wasn't gaining weight, she was happy. And if she was happy, I was ecstatic.

It wasn't as hard as you think to be on them for years. My doctors gave them to me like they were candy. To be fair, I jumped around from doctor to doctor (which is illegal, by the way, so don't do it!). I had a variety of sources. I would only have to mention that I was on them and the physicians would readily prescribe more. That's how I was able to take them for more than a decade.

While I was on and off "the scripts" in my 20's, I was fairly consistent with them in my 30's, until I hit age 37. That's when one morning I broke out in hives after taking my regular daily dose.

I knew deep down inside that it was the pills but Fat Girl assured me it was an allergic reaction to the laundry detergent, lotion, food, or anything but the pills. And I convinced myself that it was such, so I changed my eating habits, laundry detergent, and upgraded my lotion.

But my body couldn't take the abuse any more. The fact that my hair was falling out should have been an indication that something was amiss. My bangs were getting shorter and shorter. My hairstyle transformed from a sexy, side swoop to a bowl-cut mullet. But Fat Girl and I continued to ignore the elephant in the room.

I should have heeded the signs long before that morning I had hives spreading all over my supple skin. At this point, I had not only had a steady diet of prescription pills, but Fat Girl convinced me I also had to slip in some OTC appetite suppressants.

The prescription diet pills gave me pounding heart palpitations, because a lot of these pills have caffeine that ramps up your metabolism. The sound of my heart throbbing in my chest made me extremely paranoid, but that didn't stop me from taking them.

Fat Girl and I came to the conclusion that if I took the pill before work and kept myself extremely busy, I wouldn't notice all the throbbing and I would get a shitload of work done.

One particular afternoon while pecking away at my

computer, talking on the phone, and flipping through a magazine, the minor heart palpitations began to transform into a pounding in my chest, getting louder and louder.

It's like I could feel my face shake. I immediately stopped typing and stared into the computer screen waiting for my body to fall lifelessly to the floor. I asked Fat Girl "Is this it?" Thoughts of my family and daughter raced through my mind. Oh no, not here. Not at work. I could see myself being wheeled into the ambulance.

I grabbed my purse and ran to the car. I thought if I rushed to my doctor's office fast enough, they could save me. On the way, I called my mom. "Pray for me please," I told her. "I'm on my way to the doctor's office. I'm having a heart attack."

I arrived at the office and reiterated what I told them over the phone. "I'm experiencing some symptoms of a heart attack." After seeing the doctor, being hooked up to an EKG machine, and receiving a clean bill of health, I headed home early enough to hit the gym and get an early start on the evening.

Sadly, this experience was one of many. I look back and all I can do now is laugh at how ridiculous I was to rush myself to hospital ERs from Ohio to Florida, at one time or another, because I was sure that this was the big one. All in the name of skinny!

The look on the triage nurse's face when I ran into the ER and told her I was having a heart attack was one that I will never forget. But the over-exaggerated and foolish experience never stopped me from continuing to make a fool out of myself or taking diet pills.

Each time I was fine and Fat Girl was always there to confirm that the pills were harmless. We had to stay on the weight-loss plan. She'd say, "See I told you. Nothing to worry about."

Today, I think I'm done with any over-the-counter or prescription "weight-loss solution." The last diet pill I took, just a harmless product from a health and nutrition store, made me break out in a bad rash on my arms and legs.

It was a loud and clear message from my body, saying that it's done with my quick-fix, weight-loss pills. It wasn't that the product was defective. My body simply can't take any more manipulation of my fat cells and digestive system.

While waiting for my steroids prescription to be filled to handle my latest attempt at "fixing" myself, I realized that I had tried temporary fixes for years without any lasting results—which by the way is a constant letdown.

It had thrown me into a depression mode where all I could wonder about was my next weight fix: Where was it?

As I came off the diet-pill roller coaster, I could clearly see that while the diet pills helped from time to time, I was never really overweight. Even most of that pregnancy weight came off after a year.

But Fat Girl was ruthless:

- "Look at that muffin top."

- "You got a FOPA."

- "If you would just stick to the pills this wouldn't be a problem."

- "Why is it that other women can do this but you always seem to fail?"

- "You have to get rid of the fat and get it out of your system."

- "You don't have regular bowel movements like a normal person, so the fat is just going to multiply if you don't do something about it."

- "Do you just want to be fat all your life?"

She was ruthless and relentless, but I believed she just wanted the best for me. Fat Girl and I had to find a solution to get the fat out of my system and slim down.

She would say mean things to me that I accepted as fact. Hateful words like FAT and UGLY echoed loudly in my head for so long until that day I finally stopped and listened to the rest of my body, which was crying out for relief.

Relief from the appetite suppressants, and relief from the negativity I was constantly feasting on. And most of all, relief from this perpetually ugly feeling that I was fat and unattractive, with a twisted affirmation that life only begins with weight loss.

CHAPTER 6

"Get out the fat," Fat Girl would say. "Get the fat out of your FOPA. Get rid of the waste in your body. Could cleaner intestines equate to a smaller waist? What could we ingest that would not send us to the hospital AND help get rid of the fat in my digestive system?"

Fat Girl and I began to research teas and cleansers to find yet another diet avenue for weight loss. We searched out diet tricks that would manipulate my digestive system we could expel more waste (i.e., poop) from my body.

"No more bloated feeling," the products promised. "Lose 5 pounds in a week and eat whatever you want." "Get our skinny on and feel lighter." Fat Girl and I hitched our FOPA to the diet tea and cleanser bandwagon for weight loss.

Okay ladies, I'm about to get really honest here. It's unfortunate that I'm the kind of person who has a bowel movement every other day to every three days. It's pure jealousy for me to hear about people who can eat and go right to the bathroom. I've heard about these "regular" people and their daily constitutionals and their satisfaction of not being bloated.

The idea of not feeling fat and bloated sounded wonderful to Fat Girl and me. We had the same excitement as we when we saw the shake-your-fat-off-weight-loss machine. Just get regular and we are free!

If you're serious about dieting via the waste-management method, you've probably heard of or tried various versions of my favorite: Super Double Duper Dieter's Tea. If these herbal brews were able to make me regular, then I was bound and determined to map out every public bathroom within a 10-mile radius.

Fat Girl and I were in! Watch out Skinnyland, we were on our way!!

After reading several online reviews about detox herbal tea concoctions, we knew these teas were a sure answer to eliminating my FOPA. The word laxative is from the Latin word "laxus" which means to loosen. This is true from my experience, because the stimulants in the teas loosen that special muscle in your bowels at a time when you need it the most!! It's an important statement that is conveniently printed in small type on the left side of the box.

Fat Girl and I began to obsess with teas so much that we incorporated in into our daily routine. While most people were waking up to morning coffee to awaken their senses, we patiently watched the teabag steep in hot water and magically turn into a liquid FOPA eliminator.

After years (yes, years) of drinking "ignite-your-constitutional" teas, I've had some side effects that aren't conveniently listed on the side of the box. For example:

- Developing a sweat mustache and beads of sweat on your forehead while having a conversation with a coworker

- Stomach cramps and uncontrollable gas that contorts your body into unknown shapes

- Developing chicken skin goose-bumps as a notification that it's time to make power moves to the nearest bathroom

- Or best of all, having an actual volcanic-ass explosion.

Embarrassing, yet true, there were volcanic-ass experiences. After having lunch with my boyfriend one afternoon, Fat Girl and I headed back to work after taking her advice to not make a pit stop in the bathroom before leaving the apartment.

"We'll be fine. We drank the tea 4 hours ago." Fat Girl had a way with words and her advice was good as gold. During our drive, I began to feel my stomach making weird popping and squeaking sounds unlike no other sound I've ever heard before.

As we traveled through each stoplight, the sounds got louder and more intense. I thought to myself, I have more than enough time to make it back to work.

It was like an outer body experience. I could see myself helplessly losing the sphincter fight. My hands gripped the steering wheel tighter and tighter, and I started lifting my ass off the seat to get a better grip on my relaxed muscles. I shouted, "Oh no, no, NOOO!" No matter what preventative measures I took, I lost the fight.

There I was, pulled off to the side of the road; sitting

in my car in a pile of shit. "Really, Fat Girl?! Did I seriously just shit my pants?!" Of course, she didn't answer. I was alone, just me and my shit wondering what to do next.

I knew I had to head home, so I called my boyfriend and informed him to leave the apartment. I headed back. He was skeptical as to why I was coming back. "Sexy surprise," he pondered. "You just can't get enough of my sweet kisses."

It was not the time for coy answers or sexual innuendos. I plainly told him to get out of the house immediately and not to come back until I called. When I pulled into my parking space, I wondered how the hell I was going to get my ass out of the car. I thought it was a good thing I didn't wear a thong that day.

I would have to throw away my favorite, stretchy skirt that I was wearing. What could I do with a long, stretchy, black skirt? Side note that if you tie it up on both sides, it will hold everything in until you make it to the bathroom.

So there I was, walking up the stairs with a makeshift diaper on, full of shit, and moving like the Tin Man.

As I tiptoed into the house trying not to make a mess, I glanced up to find my wonderful boyfriend standing on the balcony like a knight in shining armor waiting to lend a helping hand. He must have wanted to comfort me, hearing my panicked tone over the phone.

At the same time he opened the door, I shouted,

"Don't fucking come in here!" His perplexed face turned into a sour face at the stench. He knew. And at my direction, he shut the door and turned his back.

I could try to fully elaborate the ultimate humiliation on fumigating the apartment, bagging up my shitty clothes, or swatting away flies as I scrubbed my car seat in 100 degree Florida weather, but I'm sure you get the picture. And if you're wondering, Fat Girl's after-the-fact condescending contribution to this episode was, "I bet we lost another pound! Only 9 more to go!!"

Let me assure you…there are better ways to lose weight than putting yourself at risk of losing bodily control like that! And I've been on countless teas cleansers and laxative elixirs. Super Duper Dieter's Tea (my favorite), stool softeners, prune juice, Epsom salt, Ballerina Tea, master cleanse, apple cider vinegar, lemons, colon cleansers, 7-day cleansers, 5-day cleaners, and 2-day cleansers.

You're bound to lose a pound or two, but it doesn't make you thinner. What it really does is limit the life you can lead. Besides the occasional gut-wrenching cramps, facial sweats, horrible gagging taste, loose farts, and back-fire of bloating, you will eventually succumb to your bowels becoming a ticking time-bomb on the verge of a toxic-waste disaster that limits you to a 10-mile safe radius (if you're lucky).

I look back on some of my cleanser incidents that should be untold stories taken to my grave, but all I can do now is shake my head and smile.

CHAPTER 7

You've heard it everywhere you go: eat this one thing;
consume less of this; eat more of that. Eat five small
meals a day; portions should be the size of the palm of
your hand; don't eat past 7 p.m.; high–protein is king;
no carbs; no Trans fat; low calories; no sugar; and

whatever the hell else dieticians say! Do all of this and you'll get that sublime summertime body! You've heard it, right?

You're up late watching the infomercials of the latest eating scheme cooked up in what might as well have been a diet Meth lab. You see the beautiful bodies and hear those words enticing you to transform all or just one part of your body.

It sounds so simple. I had been doing unofficial diets (no sugar this week, no dairy this a month, no carbs on the weekend, nothing white next Monday, etc.) throughout my dieting life.

In my 30's, I heard my then boss tell me about this new low-carb, diet that was all the rage. It was guaranteed to provide a full-body transformation and reform my overall eating habits. But like my boss, most people only focus on the first 14 days of the low-carb diet.

After Fat Girl and I printed out the necessary list of foods, we jumped on the low-carb bandwagon. It seemed effortless after reading about the induction phase: meat and veggies with no caffeine. It sounded like the lifestyle diet my body needed.

I learned I could have any type of meat and vegetable I wanted, but in exchange I had to give up sugar, carbs, wine, starchy foods, and fruit. Parting with my Merlot for 14 days was unheard of, but if that's what it would take to lose the FOPA, then a Merlot sacrifice it would be.

It worked too. By having less glucose to metabolize, my body focused on my stored body fat (otherwise residing in my FOPA) to create energy. Finally, the perfect diet! I could almost see Skinnyland. I had finally arrived!

Those wonderful low-carb experts who created this diet call the first phase ketosis (should call it halitosis). We all know about this phase: Your breathe stinks to high hell and tastes like dirty pennies. Of course, every diet has its ups and downs.

I called my low-carb diet plan the "Crackhead-Merlot-Monster Diet" because at the time I was craving sugar, carbs, and alcohol like it was nobody's business! I had the zombie morning breathe to prove it—24 painful hours a day for 14 long days.

Yes, low-carb diets help you lose 10 pounds (even 20 pounds, some say) in 14 days as you go through the diet's first phase. I looked and felt great as the pounds were falling off, but couldn't hold a personal conversation for the fear of seeing the other person's face melt and eyebrows fall off from the stench of my breath.

From the low-carb diet plan, Fat Girl and I went to the low-carb cooking diet plan. This cooking plan is similar to the low-carb diet but it requires you to cook using a long list of ingredients (who does that anymore?).

We thought this could be the next step for my thin-

session so I bought my diet book from secondhand store and gave it a go. Yes, I said secondhand store. It's the diet-book graveyard, selling books from people who have lost the diet-fad fight and moved on to another quick-fix. After Fat Girl informed me I could lose up to a zillion pounds in the first phase, we were all in!

The low-carb diet was easy to follow. All I had to do was go to the grocery store and pick up a head of lettuce and a rotisserie chicken. That's all I would eat all day, all the time.

The low-carb cooking plan seemed healthier but with time-consuming recipes that called for blah, blah, blah, blah! If only there was a Merlot Diet. Fun, full of happy hour laughs, easy-to-follow drinking directions, making you feel hella-sexy skinny with a slight buzz!

Both diets were helpful tools in my FOPA battle, but they never turned out to be the weight-loss salvation Fat Girl and I hoped for. With any diet that changes your eating habits over a short period of time, you know your ass will spread like melted butter once you sink your teeth into any food not listed on the matchbox-cover-sized grocery list.

But I must say the diets worked! In 14 days, I was 10 pounds thinner. However, you gain that weight back in two bites and a swallow (Like, what the hell just happened?) as soon as you start eating normal again.

One small coffee creamer, a dash of my favorite mozzarella cheese, or a scoop of sour cream and out comes the FOPA. Pop a few strawberries in my mouth? My thighs would start to wiggle with extra fluid.

Oh yeah, my thighs are the second most hated area on my body. I've had countless days when my thighs rub together enough to make my summer shorts scrunch up my ass, starting a skin-flint fire that feels like volcanic lava burning a hole in my legs.

It was insane and frustrating. I did the damn low-carb diet 15 times off and on over 5 years and I can tell you it's hard to keep up. I know the low-carb conglomeration have released new diets that are supposed to offer more nutrients and options, but restrictive eating is restrictive eating.

Eventually, you're going to want to tear down those restrictions and have that one piece of birthday cake or buttered roll at dinner without feeling enormously guilty. Wow, the two words that Fat Girl has etched into my mind: enormous and guilty. Both words I feel will never go away.

If you're anything like Fat Girl (my personal diet guru), you've likely dabbled in some of the more extreme diets like master cleanse and other cleansers I mentioned in the previous chapter.

Fat Girl even convinced me into eating a grapefruit for breakfast, lunch, and snack, and only eating a small salad for dinner. She promised that grapefruits would suppress my appetite and dissolve the fat in the FOPA.

After several weeks of scheduled workouts and consuming what seemed like a small grapefruit tree, I noticed a few nasty looking pimples on my face. Fat Girl assured me it was stress or my hormones. "Nothing to worry about." As the weeks churned on, those few pimples manifested into a full on acne convention I looked as if I was auditioning for an acne infomercial.

Next stop dermatologist, where Fat Girl and I were promptly informed that the acid from the grapefruit was not only eating the fat in the FOPA but was also creating small puss filled volcanic eruptions on my face. Fat Girl and I waited for the doctor to finish writing the prescription for what would be an embarrassing paste that had to be slather of my face three times a day.

By the way that means no makeup so I appeared to be constantly covered in sunscreen. Oh well it didn't matter because we had already began strategizing our next solution that would surely be the perfect diet that would instantly transform us into slim, trim, sexy diva!

That was the cabbage soup diet. This is straight-up cabbage soup—24/7 for seven days.

You'll lose up to 10 pounds (surprise, surprise, another 10 pound weight-loss plan) and possibly part of your dignity in the process because of the tremendous amount of uncontrollable gas fumes.

So you think you can eat only cabbage soup for seven days because you enjoy corn beef and cabbage on St. Patrick's Day?

Well this ain't your typical corn-beef-and-cabbage-holiday celebration. It's a stringy, smelly, cabbage soup that you can't entirely mask with spices.

Fuck the air fresheners and plug-ins; the smell of cabbage boiling on the stove is a constant smell of farts throughout your house and often the neighborhood.

When you open the fridge to retrieve the oversized pot of magical witches' weight-loss brew or warm up a hot steamy bowl in the microwave, you're sure to have the A de' Toilet of Cabbage. That's what Fat Girl loved to call it to encourage me to make it through another cabbage-soup consumption day.

Depending on the day, you might get to eat vegetables or fruit. But there are no other liquid except water or unsweetened fruit juice (on days when fruit is allowed).

The first two days go by okay but it's really Day Four that starts to get you. You can't put another mouthful of that gnarly cabbage soup in your mouth without involuntarily gagging.

The beauty behind the cabbage soup is that it's low-caloric food. So you can eat as much as you want without gaining weight. In what felt like never-ending days in the diet, I found myself wanting to vomit at the thought of preparing another bowl and swallowing spoonfuls of limp, tasteless leaves.

I resisted until Fat Girl forced me to crawl into the kitchen and eat the horrendous brew in hopes of losing another pound.

What the Wizards of Smart who dreamed up this diet didn't mention is that a diet of just cabbage soup, with the occasional fruit and vegetable, gives you gas. Big time!

When I say gas, I mean tremendously loud cannon farts that smell like a herd of skunks, or silent ones that sneak up and knock you out like chloroform. I've never had such bad flatulence than when I was on this diet for one week.

And I don't know one woman who ever wanted to increase their gassiness (we're not proud to fart, in public or private)!

By the end of this diet I felt weak and nauseous at the smell of cabbage soup. My knees would buckle as I walked into the kitchen for another bowl. I'm sure all the salt I poured on the soup to make it bearable didn't help my sodium levels. Yet another reason why the cabbage soup diet isn't my diet plan of choice.

Then again, I'm not really sure any diet plan has actually helped me in the long run. But one thing I'm 100% sure of is that I will never eat another piece of cabbage in my entire life. I don't care if it was sautéed, fried, baked, or wrapped in bacon!

I say to you, these lips will never grace cabbage again! Not even coleslaw!

And that's the thing to take away from diets—they aren't a long-term weight-loss solution. You can drop those 10 pounds in two weeks. But beyond those 10 pounds, your weight loss will plateau and stop.

Plus, it's a hard to keep up the enthusiasm for a bland or restricted diet. You will start to question why you're really putting yourself through the aggravation and misery of crawling to the kitchen for another bubbling bowl of liquid gas.

CHAPTER 8

If you watch enough late-night TV, you eventually
make your way to those lovely infomercials where
some 20-something with abs of steel is scantily clad

and telling you that you can look just like her (or him) if you do this one exercise system for 6 weeks (3 months, 1 year, forever, whatever the fine print says).

And when I say scantily clad, I mean she's wearing short–ass shorts, has zero body fat, and is pleasantly smiling because she's a 19-year-old fitness model and has no damned idea what it's like to have a FOPA. Really?!

If I sound like I'm jealous that's because I AM. What I would give up to have just one exercise day in my spandex shorts turning heads instead of having said shorts roll down underneath my belly with every painful movement.

But what do we do after hearing that we too can achieve these amazing results? We buy the damned exercise system, of course!

I've been in the video workout world for decades. I can still remember wanting to look like Jane Fonda with the awesome leg warmers and cool workout clothes. Fat Girl and I were on a mission to find a workout that would help me pull those stomach muscles back together, shed my FOPA, and have abs so tight I could wash my panties on them!

After Jack La Lane and Jane Fonda, Fat Girl and I began our quest into the workout world from VHS to DVD. We were bound to transform my body into that of a fit, workout-video vixen.

To be honest, I was an active participant of the black

market or bootlegged workout DVDs. Desperate times call for desperate and cheap measures. After not making it through the warm up and sitting on the couch watching the last 45 minutes, with a glass of Merlot, I was glad I didn't skip paying the electric bill in exchange for the easy 3 payments of $49.95, plus shipping and handling.

But every time a new fitness craze came out, Fat Girl's voice was loud, clear, and repetitive in my head: "You've got to try it, this is the one!"

We were workout video junkies. If I couldn't make it through a difficult video then we were off to the next one. Slim in 10, 15 or 20, International Butt Lift, Choose a Letter – Number, Yoga for Beginners, Insanely Painful, Latin Dance, Jane Fonda collection, and even those brutal militant bootcamp DVDs

The list goes on and on. I loved them all for one reason or another. I'd try these exercise tapes and jump right into the lunges, Pilates, squats, crunches, and other calisthenics. I've even searched the Internet for short homemade workouts from women like myself in the FOPA Fight.

Accessories are a must. I've since graduated from using canned vegetables and gallon water bottles as weights. I currently own a Bosu ball, exercise ball, dumbbells, kettle bell, yoga mats, blocks, ankle weights, iron weights, plastic weights, hand bands, rubber bands (that thing that goes around your thighs), belts (waist trainer and the sweat belt), suspension lines, and other workout gear that promised to help me get slim.

I'm sorta stuck on workout videos but they all work to some extent—if you get through them. You can drop two pants sizes, but that's usually because you're in traction from pulling a muscle that you didn't know you had and your jaw is wired shut after you passed out and fell on your face while trying to do a downward dog!

Every time I saw one of those infomercials convincing me that I could indeed have killer abs with just 6 minutes of work, I would get an adrenaline rush. It was the shake-your-fat-off machine all over again. Needless to say, Fat Girl and I were all in. "Just get through this set of DVD's for 6 weeks and you'll be all set. Skinnyland, here we come!"

Let's get real. There is a little difference between full-on cardiac arrest and getting six pack abs. Fat Girl reassured me that I could do it but getting my ass into the groove of starting these kick-ass cardio workout routines was another story.

It usually took me a good two weeks to work up the nerves to open the package and start the video. I remembered the pains that would give a drill sergeant goose bumps.

That's not to say you never get positive results, but it's not instantaneous or without significant effort (and in some cases, pain). I think it would be more effective if the case read, "This DVD workout will painfully kick your ass into shape."

Don't get me wrong. I love, love, love the workout DVDs. But they are a lot of work. With most sessions, I thought I was going to pass out.

And since I have no rhythm, I felt like I was working twice as hard to keep up with the instructors and those little sweaty, smiling assistants. The thought of me performing a hip-hop routine with my arms flying in the air, gyrating my hips horrendously off beat, but feeling like I'm a dancing queen is mostly effective.

I can honestly say that these workouts are very hard. I can still feel the clicking in my jaw from hitting myself in the face with an upper cut!! No pain, no gain!

Fat Girl lured me to the gym with the promise of a free consultation from a personal trainer. Our trainer looked similar to the Incredible Hulk, with a bouffant that had long ponytail attached.

We were certain that his pleasant, soft voice would provide us with a soothing FOPA-illuminating workout. Little did we know that we were about to embark on a dumbbell, squat, push-up, jumping jack, crunch, extravaganza that I can only compare to medieval torture.

Upon conclusion of the workout, our pleasant voice instructor asked if he could schedule us for an ongoing workout program. I was unable to speak. I could see his mouth moving but all I could think about was why is the room spinning.

I don't think I answered. I just remember looking in the mirror and noticing that one arm was shorter that the other. As I kicked my gym bag to the parking lot towards my car all I could think was who's going to drive me home because I can't feel my arms.

I've also done the boot-camp sessions. You know— those outdoor exercise classes where you're pretty convinced you're going to throw up a lung because you have never been forced to do so many push-ups, leg lifts, lunges, and sprints outside in the 100 degree Florida weather.

You feel better once you're done and forget most of the pain until the next class. So when the instructor has you running around the parking lot, you fantasize about running to your car and driving over him.

I even went to a trainer when I didn't have the money to spare. I was going to the Dominican Republic and Fat Girl convinced me I needed to go all out to look good for my vacation. The trainer worked out my back to make it smaller so I had a higher butt and tiny waist.

It was great until I went on vacation to an all-inclusive resort. As a reward, Fat Girl and I ate pretty much everything on the island. We came home happy and heavy, and never went back to the trainer. But I must admit I was really sexy for about a week.

I won't lie. Fat Girl remains diligent at making sure I never forget the feeling of that 9-year-old girl standing in the dining room that Sunday evening so long ago.

Fat Girl asks some tough questions before, during, and after workouts:

- "Why do you have clothes that you can't fit into?"

- "Isn't it painful when you sit down and your stomach hangs over your pants??"

- "Why is it that every time you take off your jeans you have a button imprint on your gut and pocket whelps on your ass?"

- "Aren't you tired of being fat?"

I can't stop those thoughts from popping in my head but my hope is to avoid going through the desperation cycle I've clung to with past exercise regimens and take on something that's more successful this go-around.

CHAPTER 9

You might have had a similar experience but here is how those workout programs have been for me:

1   You start the workout program and put in a hard effort for the first four days.

2   You're sore because your body isn't used to the exertion and you think that those body aches should equate to substantial results. (Nobody is there to tell you that achy muscles are just the start to a fit and healthy body.)

3   You get up the next morning and weigh yourself. You don't see the results you want so you get depressed and sometimes give up.

It's a letdown and a sure path to failure if you let that happen. What we want to push aside is the old adage that it takes discipline and consistent effort to reshape your body.

Plus, there are a million other things you could be doing with your time—like having a glass of wine and watching a good movie to let your mind unwind after a long day at work.

Many times, I would start a workout like T-25 and feel on top of the world because the exercises don't seem that bad if you do them one time. But have you held a squat for a minute after you've been working hard? There is some serious wobbling and shaking from your toes to your teeth and you're convinced this is the beginning of spontaneous combustion.

The concept of short workouts are so appealing when

you start but sticking with the program day after day without the results is what kills the drive to continue. I would get up and allow Fat Girl to set the tone for the day by zoning in on that one body flaw I was hoping I could change with exercise.

And she was vicious: "Your boobs are sagging. You have back fat. Your arms are jiggling. There are dimples on your butt. Your FOPA is sticking out more than yesterday."

You keep hoping these flaws will go away and when they don't, it's unbearable. You want change to happen quickly but there's no set timeframe when it comes to your body and weight loss.

You're unique. You have a different metabolism, digestive system, exercise effort, and desire from that of other people. Trainers can say your body will change within six weeks of working out (along with healthier eating) but realistically it could take longer. They also point out that it's 80 percent healthy eating and 20 percent regular high-intensity exercise that influence weight loss.

But again, that's hard to internalize and believe when that yearning to get outside of this current body you don't love is so terribly strong. You feel panic and anxiety. It's what spurs you to try other exercises that promise quicker results.

I don't totally believe it yet, but I am starting to accept that nothing can provide you a quick fix when it comes to a fit body. Fat Girl still says its right around the corner.

Good fitness takes constant work. It's something that requires regular maintenance and upkeep, just as you would paint your house to keep it looking good or get your car's oil changed to have it running reliably.

But that yearning to have a different body is what Fat Girl tells me about all the time…and she beats me up with the negativity for not having that "perfect body."

CHAPTER 10

I think I'm slightly brave enough to try new techniques and methods to get rid of the FOPA but medical procedures make me extremely nervous and more importantly are way beyond my budget.

But that's not to say that Fat Girl and I haven't looked

into various procedures to tighten the abs, smooth out the cellulite, and suck out the fat.

Several times throughout the day, Fat Girl and I surf the Internet for surgical, before-and-after weight-loss photos. I felt a connection with these nameless and faceless women with body parts very similar to mine.

I could relate to their frustrations of desperately wanting to achieve the perfect self-image, wear a bikini, or just feel comfortable in their clothes. They were also underwater, wanting to reach the top and finally take a breath just like me.

The constant reading of patient reviews, doctor recommendations, and best of all the after photos were exhilarating. The outstanding pictures of successful results reminded us of the shake-your-fat-off machine once again.

The procedures were way beyond my miniscule paycheck and weak credit for the easy-approved payment plan. But Fat Girl was determined there was a perfect procedure out there for us and the search was on.

We found free consultations and discount coupons for lunchtime lipo, body wraps, cool lasers, hot lasers, tummy tucks, awake lipo, asleep lipo, twilight lipo, you name it…we found it! There were procedures that can suck, melt, cut, stitch, tuck, freeze, heat, cool, or fry the fat off any part of your body.

With the strong encouragement from Fat Girl, we went

to an appointment that would freeze my FOPA into a liquid that would secrete through my lymph nodes.

Did I mention that cancer runs rampant in my family and I'm pretty sure I'm gonna need those lymph nodes later? Fat Girl ignored my concerns after the nurse stated the liquid was the size of a French fry and harmless.

The consultation ended like all the others: a pretty folder with an enormous estimate minus a FOPA-eliminating procedure appointment.

All the doctor visits resulted in wasted gas and time. To our surprise, the discount coupon for most procedures only covered the small section below my belly button. What about the other half of my FOPA, above my belly button? And the love handles? And the other fat sections of my body?

There had to be an at-home technique or procedure that didn't require a medical license, using equipment I could purchase from the local pharmacy. I heard horror stories of women reverting to unlicensed individuals who pretended to be physicians and performed procedures in their homes. Well, I can say this. Fat Girl would never get me to cross that road.

But home remedies and procedures had Fat Girl and me curious. And they were damn convincing, especially the vapor-rub-and-plastic-wrap fat vaporizing treatment.

It was quite interesting to and did I mention cheap!!!

The technique called for vapor rub and plastic wrap. The blog had several positive reviews, which excited Fat Girl and me into running to the store right after work so we could be part of the success stories.

After returning from the store, I was anxiously awaiting the results of my overnight transformation. I had it all planned out: rub it on, wrap it up, sleep, and I'd wake up with 2 inches of FOPA vaporized. I would be looking and feeling sexy by morning!

The thought of my body after performing this technique for 4 weeks had Fat Girl saying, "Sexy thongs, here we come!"

I was set, laying comfortably in bed, and dozing off into my skinny dreams. It felt good. I was relaxed. I could feel a little tingling here and there but Fat Girl assured me it was just the cool tingling from the vapor rub. "It's working."

So I slept, but not for long. About 15 minutes into my REM sleep stage, my eyes and mouth opened. I think Fat Girl screamed because nothing came out of my mouth. I asked Fat Girl, "Was the fire alarm going off?" "Is my bed on fire?"

She was speechless. And then it hit me. My freaking FOPA was on fire—literally being vaporized!

I ran into the bathroom. I couldn't get the waist trainer and plastic wrap off fast enough. It felt as though the unraveling of plastic lasted forever.

I just knew I'd end up in another embarrassing emergency room visit. I could see myself standing there with my stomach burned off explaining to the same ER nurse…it was just vapor rub and plastic wrap.

Thankfully, I was fine. Just a little disappointed at another failed fat reduction attempt. Fat Girl was also disappointed and still unsatisfied. "Our solution is out there. And we're going to find it."

CHAPTER 11

In addition to all the techniques and eating plans, I also
joined weight-loss support programs. One in particular
that I attended at the YMCA was very memorable. It
was my safe haven, a room full of women who knew

exactly how I felt and were also in need of eliminating their FOPAs.

I loved the group; it was a sisterhood. Women gathered together for the common good or bad, which was our FAT.

I really enjoyed discussing my eating and exercising obstacles with women who also struggled with their own Fat Girls. We talked, we shopped for diet powdered foods and shakes, and we paid our dues at the end of our weekly meetings.

The best part of the meetings was the success stories and the administering of stickers for people hitting their weekly weight-loss targets. It was awesome. I was all in, 100% dedicated to eating the bland foods and bitter desserts accompanied by a regimented exercise routine.

Around the fourth week during the sticker award ceremony, Fat Girl whispered, "What the heck are you clapping for? You haven't gotten any stickers since we've started!"

As I looked around the room to see the cheers of the other women with their badges of honor, I realized they were winning. They were all winning and I hadn't been winning or getting any stickers.

I felt like the wind had been knocked out of me. How could this be? Fat Girl and I were certain that it had to be our food intake so we decided to eat less, and work out more. Fat Girl was confident that adjustments in my point plan would be the answer to losing the weight and getting the sticker recognition that we deserved.

After two more weeks of paying dues and increased cardio workouts, I was sure that the next meeting would be the one. Finally, winning!

The meeting started off as always with discussions of new food products (more "yummy" flavorless foods and powdered drinks) and minutes of the last meeting. Fat Girl and I were anxious and ready to hear the applause and stand proudly as I received my shiny sticker.

But I ended up speechless. I hid my disappointment behind a big goofy grin as I stepped off the scale and realized my weight-loss disappointment. I gained two pounds. Our minor adjustments to the perfect point plan failed. Fat Girl was more than furious as she spewed words of self-hatred while I watched others winning the battle of the bulge.

Our plan for the next meeting was foolproof. Increase the workouts and follow the eating plan to the T. But the anxiety of gaining more weight and not making the cut in the next meeting was unbearable. The flashbacks of that fateful Sunday afternoon began to consume me. And the chants of Fat Girl repeated in my head. "You just can't fail again! Must you humiliate yourself every time?"

I just couldn't bring myself to step on the scale. My palms were sweating and I felt the knots in my stomach. I couldn't bring myself to attend another meeting and not get any stickers. So I did what any self-respecting person would do. I went to the dollar store and bought my own damn stickers! Fat Girl and I had our award ceremony complete with Merlot, fish taco sliders, and shiny new stickers!

I knew there was a weight-loss program to help me locate my perfect self-image and eliminate my FOPA. Maybe not the meetings at the YMCA but I knew it was out there in diet world.

So much so that Fat Girl and I began the road to acupuncture. Like I said before, I'm not one for medical procedures or needles. But after a quick 3-minute consultation, Fat Girl and I were all in, once again!

It turned out to be not as bad as I thought. Not painful but quite weird. The doctor was an extremely polite, young physician who liked to discuss his failing love life, overbearing mother, and plans to take a year off to live in Paris.

The conversation was entertaining but all I could think about was the cellulite that was escaping my body with each prick of the needle like a deflating balloon.

In addition to my acupuncture appointments, Fat Girl was adamant that we keep on our regimented workout schedule: DVD workouts during the week, cardio on Saturday, and acupuncture twice a week. It seemed to be working by the comments of "your beginning to get buffed" from my acupuncturist. Fat Girl and I were elated.

The conversations got a bit more personal. We discussed our hopes, dreams, daily routines, and more stories of failing relationships. I figured if the doctor was enjoying my visits and providing FOPA eliminating solutions, it was a win-win with Fat Girl and me. The doctor suggested adding B-12 shots and mermaid exercises. Yes, I said mermaid exercises.

I thought for a moment is this some kind of joke. As I shook my head in agreement with doing the new exercises, I politely asked him to demonstrate. Fat Girl and I felt the adrenaline pulsing through our veins. It was the fat-shaking-machine all over again. We waited with anticipation.

He sat on the chair, leaned back, and began performing stomach crunches alternating his legs at an angle. Really? That's it?!

It was the shake-your-fat-off machine (all bark and no bite). But that didn't stop Fat Girl and me from performing the awkward workout move before jumping in the shower for work. The acupuncturist was thin and this secret exercise took him to Thinville. It was sure to work for me to.

During one of my appointments, as the soft music played and thoughts of me running topless on the beach ran through my head, I felt a small twitch of my thumb. I said to myself or rather to Fat Girl, "What was that?"

I lay stone still, waiting for the next twitch. It happened again and again. I began to position my arm to reach for the emergency alert button. As I reached for the device, my thumb and first finger stiffened like a board.

The turning of my head made the acupuncture pin in my forehead feel numb and the view of the alert device was lost from the acupuncture pins protruding from my face. I was a human pin cushion.

I began to panic and my heart started racing. I'm paralyzed. Oh no. I asked Fat Girl "What about my daughter?" "Was becoming paralyzed worth it?" Fat Girl was silent.

As the last resort ran through my mind of flopping onto the tile floor and bleeding to death from the acupuncture needles in popped the doctor with a smile. I was greatly relieved. He removed the needles and I politely left face and fingers twitching without making another appointment.

CHAPTER 12

What's probably the most amazing and saddest part of my multi-decade diet is the amount of control I have given to Fat Girl to dictate the terms of how I lived my life. I turned down opportunities in my life that could have been beneficial for me and my daughter, and created fear that prevented me from ever knowing failure or success.

So much time wasted, all in the name of FAT.

Fat Girl was always more than obliged to remind me, "You're too out of shape to be successful." Looking back on all I've put my body through, the psychological mind games and refined self-fear I've created, I guess it could be an addiction of sorts.

I'm not sure. It's one thing to state I'm going to conquer this epic mental fat battle than to actually put a plan into action. My mother always says and still does say, "If you only saw the beautiful person everyone else sees."

If only I could change the thought process that has prevented me from knowing the authentic me.

I've always had the support of friends and a prayerful family that prevented me from implementing any fatal plan when my fat-inspired depression reached an all-time low.

My never-ending woes about my bulging stomach and thick thighs took their toll. My supporters' casual reply of "you're not fat" was their way of saying they wanted to move on. But those words didn't resonate with my mind. And certainly not with Fat Girl.

She knows me better than I know myself. And until we are skinny or feel some kind of self-worth, she will continue to force me into this weight-loss war. Reassurances only bolstered her conviction that I was most definitely fat and in need of a new fix.

I went along with her suggestions because no matter

what my weight really was, I felt fat. I felt claustrophobic, unable to breathe, and stuck in a body that I didn't want.

It's like being under water, seeing the surface, and unable to swim to the top. You want to breathe and you know when you reach the surface, you will breathe. But I feel like I'll never able to reach the surface. If only I could take that one breathe of relief.

I work to keep these irrational feelings from taking over even today, but I get to points where the panicky feelings start bubbling up to the surface. I'm not sure if this will one day subside or I will have to struggle for the rest of my life.

For right now, that desire to be outside my body is there. And I can hear Fat Girl: "You're crazy if you're going to tell yourself your body is okay right now. I know the truth. You're fat."

I don't verbally talk back to her but I do everything I can to shut those thoughts down before they pick up momentum. If I don't, there will be an avalanche effect where the direness of the situation gets me so down that I don't recover quickly. I'm stuck in that depression.

It's like you wake up and whatever you didn't like about yourself (wrinkles under your eyes or chicken wings for arms) is still there but magnified in your mind. Oftentimes, I reinforced this with the scale.

I would start off my morning, every day, weighing

myself—because of course that's the best time of the day when you haven't consumed and feel the lightest.

I haven't gotten on the scale this week because I just started working out again and I don't want to sabotage those efforts. I'm not ready for that yet.

See! That's how powerful the scale is as a determinant of my inner peace and happiness.

I know if I get on the scale and I see a number I don't like (and that's sadly most of the time) then I assume and internalize failure. Fat Girl hounds me. Even now when I have more control over my thoughts and I'm doing so much better, I know those weaknesses are there.

Like most women, I started weighing myself young, probably around the 9th grade. I was in the drill team and we had to be a certain weight. Our waist and other body parts had to fit certain measurements to wear the uniforms. A few years later when I left Ohio to go to Florida, it became a daily habit: Get up, pee, and weigh myself.

What's scary is that the scale can become addictive. You're constantly monitoring yourself, whether the weight is going up or down. Before I knew it, I started weighing myself more often than just once in the morning: When I got home; before school; after dinner; and whenever Fat Girl demanded it. I was on the scale.

I used to work at a warehouse for a while that had a

big truck scale. Yup. I used to get on that too and weigh myself to see how I was doing while working.

It was tough and I used that scale every morning to confirm Fat Girl's accusations that I was fat. I bought workout clothes and started walking every morning, but the weight was barely budging.

I would cry because I was so heavy. That was the biggest I had ever been and yet some days (many pounds lighter now) I feel exactly as I did then.

CHAPTER 13

There are some days I can't believe I let myself feel the way I do. My relationship with Fat Girl still continues but she takes into consideration that I'm older and my body will not magically transform into the after pictures we've seen on the Internet. However, I'm still carrying around a to-do list, both physically and mentally!!!

After 45 and counting diet techniques from A to Z…I still have my FOPA, which I have promised to love since it is a part of me. It's a great reminder of beginning my life as a mother.

That's a chapter of my life that I'm most proud of and my greatest accomplishment. My FOPA will always be my daughter's apartment that she leased for nine months.

My unexpected diet journey has enabled me to share my struggle with self-deprecation and bullying. I want women to know that our Creator never intended for all our curves to be identical. Our DNA and body types are our heritage, our unique life story. I've learned that every curve has its purpose, like thick hips and thighs protecting our joints.

Looking back on the mental and physical torment I put myself through has become my daily reminder that I am not perfect but I'm happy. I want to own my body and love me. I feel so much happier loving myself. Being able to feel good about yourself creates self-worth and an eagerness to live life and seek joy.

I'm not saying that I'm totally free of all self-hatred and Fat Girl. Every day is a constant struggle. But every morning, when my eyes open, is another day I'm privileged to make improvements to my life and to others.

For several months of my life I stopped looking at myself in the mirror because I was repulsed at my reflection. I let men take advantage of because I yearned for love and I thought the minor gestures of caring would fulfill the void of loving myself. I stopped loving myself and focused my attention on seeking out diets that would mold me into a fictional character that Fat Girl had led me to believe was the perfect picture of beauty.

Did you ever avoid looking at yourself in a mirror for a year because you couldn't stand what you might see?

Did you brush your teeth in a dark bathroom just to avoid seeing chubby arms or a rounded tummy?

Did you let men take advantage of your low self-esteem?

Or have negative actions or words become a part of your life like molestation, alcoholism, depression, abusive relationships, or suicide?

Have you allowed darkness to become a part of you?

Have you lost control of your life and let achievable goals escape you?

I did.

After years of Fat Girl telling me I was no good, ugly, and fat, I surrendered. I accepted incorrect labels from the time my sister uttered those hateful words that manifested into my inner Fat Girl.

How do you move forward in your career, create lasting relationships, and build a successful life when you have no self-worth? In most cases like mine, it's an everyday struggle.

It's weird because you can go to work and carry on like everything is normal, but inside you don't see yourself the way your colleagues, friends, or family member see you. It's a dark inner secret.

I can't even fully explain the self-hatred and ugliness that I allowed to brew in my mind for so many years. And I don't condone it. I searched out every bad or challenging aspect in my life and attributed it to my weight and looks. That mirror wasn't just a reflection of me...it was my own condemnation of who I was.

When you are that entirely opposed to your essence (your true being) because all you can see is the physical being in front you then the feelings that you're left with are bleak.

I can remember one afternoon, in the middle of this inner-directed rampage, talking to my girlfriend. We were outside in sunny Florida and it was a simply gorgeous day. As I looked into the beautiful blue sky, I told my girlfriend, "Today is a great day to die." That's a terrible response to a day that should have been treasured to the fullest.

I had all sorts of ideas of killing myself because I was tired of the weight battle. Thankfully, I could never bring myself to do any of them because of my daughter. I knew I couldn't be that selfish to her.

I know why I felt that way. I had allowed Fat Girl to influence me. I loathed who I was, believing that it all went back to my weight. To be clear, I had the power in me all along to fight back and stop this wave of depression.

Now that I'm older, I question my self-hatred and Fat Girl's brutality toward me. Sometimes, I wonder if she really loves me. I can't imagine saying the things she has said to someone I love. I was supposed to love myself, yet I betrayed my inner being by believing Fat Girl's negativity. And I stopped living a full life because of that.

Have you been allowing your inner negativity to talk to you this way? Do you believe that imaginary monster?

I want you to know right now that this inner negative person is LYING to you. Every word Fat Girl says is not true AND she isn't right.

That's not your true self. It's not the real you.

There are times I look back at my life and I'm filled with regret that I believed Fat Girl for so long. I have so much to offer yet I was convinced I didn't because I bought the lies of appearances.

I'm not heavy but you know there are many curvaceous women who are happy. They are in love. With themselves, in loving relationships and in their careers. They are successful moms and caretakers. They do whatever they want to do with spunk and a zest for life!

Yes, these women are out there, along with the skinny

ones we think have all the fun. But back when I was stuck in my depression, I was critical and confused of these women. Instead of celebrating them, I felt they had stolen what I wanted so desperately--but I believed I had to be thin!

When I turned 40, I started focusing on my accomplishments. In the last few years, I have started to talk back to Fat Girl.

I started doing healthier things in my life with my eating and exercising. It's nothing radical. Radical just makes you exhausted and beaten down. I made the transition mentally because I couldn't deal with any more negativity.

It's a very tedious and slow process getting to know yourself and loving who you are. I have to verbally talk myself out of negative thoughts, but that's what I do.

Last week, I was getting ready to go out to dinner and I said to my boyfriend, "I feel fat in what I have on." My boyfriend asked if I wanted to stay home. He's incredibly sweet that way (he kinda knows about my hang-ups).

But I knew that if I didn't leave the house every time I felt fat or uncomfortable I would never fucking leave the house! For some people, it comes easy and you don't have to work at it. I, however, do have to work at it, and there's nothing wrong with that.

Fat Girl will always be a part of me. But I've stripped

away her power. She's more likely to jump on my train to Happyville or at least consider getting on rather than focusing on my FOPA.

I don't want to overhype it, but there may always be the constant fear inside of me that I will become overweight. The danger of thinking this way is that you assume life is going to be perfect if you lose the weight.

You think that every problem and annoyance will be resolved. You think you're going to feel different because you look different. Your lifestyle will change and it will be a Cinderella moment.

Hmm, but what if you don't realize that you are in your Cinderella moment?

I looked at a picture of myself 3 years ago and I was amazed at how good I looked. I would kick myself in the nose if I could. But at the time, I didn't feel that way. I remember thinking my boobs are sagging. I have back fat. I have dimples on my butt. I need to get these jiggly legs tightened up.

Now, I look at that picture of a strong and beautiful woman and think if I looked that way I wouldn't complain.

At my graduation for my Master's Degree; seeing my daughter grow into a beautiful young woman; holding hands with my mother; at happy hour laughing with my girlfriends and at other times I have experienced the overwhelming feelings of love that touches the soul.

So how do you make that change in thinking?

Realize first of all that you have the inner strength to do this. The mind is an amazing and unmeasured mechanism for potential. That potential can be good or bad, depending on the focus of your thoughts.

For me, shifting the focus of my thoughts had a lot do with faith. I'm not a devout religious person, even being raised in the Baptist Church. But I think there is a spiritual being in all of us. We must find that connection and nurture it.

Of course, my family and daughter played a big role in changing my thinking. They make up my circle of love, laughing, and living. When you open your eyes and take your first breath, know that valuable moment was meant for you—because you only get one ride at life. Do you really want to waste your time?

I don't think so. I think, like me, you're a smart and beautiful woman with more to offer than you realize. The first thing to do is to acknowledge that, even when your inner voices might scream at you because of your weight (or wrinkles, or dull hair, or whatever).

Let go of whatever scary, bad, sad, hateful, disruptive, or unpleasant event that happened in the past. I can't do anything about stuff that happened two weeks ago, let alone decades ago.

But I can do something right now, in my next second

or minute, as I live in the moment and be happy. I don't have to be negative anymore. There will be bad days. That's life—our testimonies. But no more will I let them outweigh my great days.

Sometimes when I'm sitting on the couch, I grab hold of FOPA and shake it but not with the same hatred and anger as when I was much younger. Yes, the FOPA is still there although it has fluctuated in size over the years. It's still soft and mushy, and decorates my belly button.

Fat Girl's voice isn't as loud and boisterous. Her love for me is stronger than ever but she's much kinder than when I was 9. She still eagerly searches for ways to make improvements to my womanly curves. I'm positive that our diet journey will continue creating stories of success and failures.

But now I have the courage and fortitude to say no and not beat myself up or let Fat Girl beat me up. I've come to realize there is no magic cure for my FOPA; no super pill or fantasy diet.

It takes hard work, a consistent workout routine, better dietary choices, mental and spiritual growth, and an ever increasing love of self. I'm investing more in my personal trainer and dietary needs and less into Merlot.

Don't get me wrong. I'm still trying to come up with the perfect Merlot diet that will forever dissolve my FOPA but for now Fat Girl and I have decided together that it's better to be healthy, happy, and loved.

CHAPTER 14

Loving yourself isn't easy for everyone. If you're like me and have a Fat Girl—or whatever you call the negative voice in your mind—it takes daily work!!!! I have to constantly remind myself how valuable my life is, and loving me is the first step in that direction.

The following points help me stay focused on the importance of my life, being happy and healthy.

In The Morning

- It's so easy for you to-do list to pop in your mind as soon as you wake in the morning. Replace those stressful first thoughts to thankful and grateful thoughts. When I first open my eyes in the morning, I thank my Creator for blessing me with another day to better my life and the lives of those around me.

- Look at yourself in the mirror in the morning and say the things you like about yourself. For example, it helps me when I say them out loud. I usually point out all the good parts of my body while I'm brushing my teeth.

- Hang a picture of yourself on your vision board or bathroom mirror to work toward a better you I used to have a picture of a celebrity but realistically, I don't have a trainer, dietician, or fully equipped gym at my disposal and my body has gone through childbirth. I want a better me, not a better unattainable someone else. Search around Pinterest if you aren't yet at the point where you love yourself in photos.

- Add errands for a better you to your daily checklist. In addition to paying bills and getting my oil changed, I added exercise, meditation, drinking plenty of water and other important reminders that will benefit me.

During Your Day

- Make a list of great things currently happening in your life to remind yourself of your many blessings. It's easy for me to think of one negative aspect of my life and spiral into depression. Before those thoughts begin filling up in my head, I grab a pen and paper (often a sticky note) and write down my blessings as constant reminders throughout my day. Don't feel like these need to be big deals. Sometimes it's the blessing of someone holding the door open for me or getting a green light when I'm in a rush to work.

- Create a vision board but just don't list your goals. Write down the steps on how you'll reach each goal. Health, happiness, freedom are all listed on my vision board but I also list doctor's appointments, meditation time, and ways to save money to travel. Don't worry about having all the right answers. Just getting going puts you ahead of others and achieving your dreams!

- It's ok if you don't clean your plate. Times were hard when I was growing up and we were taught to always "clean your plate" and "there are children starving all over the world, you have to eat all of your food". Habits are hard to break and I find myself having to clean my plate so I always put small portions on my plate to eliminate any quilt.

Keep In Mind

- Get regular check-ups because knowing what's going on inside your body is just as important as the reflection we see in the mirror. When my physician informs me that my exams results are in good shape, I feel so much better about my eating habits and exercise.

I hope you're able to use these points to make progress. Don't forget to track your journey to Happyville!

Your Journey Journal to Happyville Begins Now:

_____
_____
_____
_____
_____
_____
_____
_____
_____
_____
_____
_____
_____
_____
_____
_____
_____
_____
_____
_____
_____
_____
_____
_____
_____
_____
_____